Created to Crave

A BIBLICAL GUIDE TO REDIRECT YOUR
DESIRES AND OVERCOME EMOTIONAL
EATING

Dr. Erica Callahan

Fose Media, LLC
Waterloo, NY

The stories in this book are based on individuals the author knows personally or professionally. To protect the privacy of those individuals, names and details have been changed.

Created to Crave / Erica Callahan. —1st ed.
ISBN 9781521245538

Disclaimer

The information provided in this book is designed to provide helpful information on the subjects discussed. This book is not meant to be used, nor should it be used, to diagnose or treat any medical condition. For diagnosis or treatment, consult your primary care provider. The publisher and author are not responsible for any specific health or allergy needs that may require medical supervision and are not liable for any damages or negative consequences from any treatment, action, application or preparation, to any person reading or following the information in this book. References are provided for informational purposes only and do not constitute endorsement of any websites or other sources. Readers should be aware that websites listed in this book may change their content after the book has been published.

Copyright Notices

Contents

Dedication

To my husband and best friend, Aaron. He calls me beautiful and brilliant.

To my mother in law, Joanne, a steadfast example of a Godly woman who serves her King with grace. She calls me precious and sweet.

And ultimately to my Lord, Savior, King and Friend. He lovingly calls me all those names and so much more.

It is my daily choice to believe them!

"For I know the plans I have for you," declares the Lord, "plans to prosper you and not to harm you, plans to give you hope and a future."

— Jeremiah 29:11 (NIV)

Introduction

You are not an accident. You are not a product of chance. You were lovingly created by a God who passionately wants a personal relationship with you.

God's Word says you are fearfully and wonderfully made (Psalm 139:14). Do you believe that? You were created for a purpose and God has a divine plan for your life.

We are handcrafted by the Creator and covered in His fingerprints. However, the corruption of sin has taken its toll on our world and on our bodies. God gave us food to satisfy and sustain us, not to stumble us.

Maybe you've asked God to take away your cravings for junk food. Maybe you've asked Him to take away your desire for that treat that you can't help reaching for when you are stressed.

I'd like to suggest that you don't need a reduced desire for junk food, you need an *increased* desire for God. Only He can satisfy. And He promises to do just that, but only if we look to Him as our Sustainer. Using food to dull the hurt or soothe the stress isn't the answer. **He is**.

There is a battle raging in your body. Your whole body is involved: mind, heart, hormones and belly. So many things influence what you put into your mouth. Your mood influences your choice of food. Your food choices influence your mood.

You need to eat to live. But is your belly having undue influence on your life? Why do you crave certain foods? How can you bring your body, mind and heart into the unity that God intended you to have? How can you win the battle for your belly?

I'll show you. I certainly don't have all the answers, but I know the One who does. I will reveal the link between your mood and food and show how hormones play a huge part in what and when you eat. I'll reveal what the Bible says about our struggle with food and I'll show you God's promises for your life.

Take heart dear sister, there is hope! You are loved more than you can ever imagine by a Father who wants nothing less for you than a healthy, joy-filled life that comes from a heart surrendered to Him.

CHAPTER 1

You're Unique!

> *You made my whole being; you formed me in my mother's body. I praise you because you made me in an amazing and wonderful way.*
>
> *- Psalm 139:13-14 (NCV)*

I take great delight in the variety of people I see in my office where I practice chiropractic and nutritional counseling. Just like snowflakes, no two of my patients are alike. They come in all shapes and sizes, all nationalities and backgrounds, and with an amazing array of quirks and temperaments.

The most wonderful aspect of working with so many people is the realization that we are not all "cookie-cutter" copies. God made us unique and has given each of us a special purpose. His purpose is accomplished through all our different personality traits, characteristics, desires, and emotions.

If you have kids, I'm sure you've experienced the embarrassment when one of them points out in public (at the top of their lungs of course!) how someone looks or acts different. Joanne told me of the time that her family stopped at a gas station to fill up. Her six-year-old son pointed to a burly motorcycle rider sporting a red mohawk and loudly proclaimed, "Mom, that man looks like a chicken!" (referring to his hair looking like that red flap that sticks out of the top of a chicken's head). Joanne was mortified and feared for her life! Thankfully, he only shot a sour look in their direction before driving off.

Seventeen years later, I married that little boy. Joanne is my mother-in-law. And my husband will never live down that story. Naturally, our seven-year-old daughter has done similar things on multiple occasions and we constantly must remind her that God made everyone different and He loves us all the same!

Take my one patient, 85-year-old Sally, for example. Sally stands tall and confident despite only being 4 foot 9 inches and weighing less than 100 pounds. With a spring in her step and twinkle in her eye, she enters the treatment room and shares how she "has smoked 10 cigarettes every day for as many years as I can remember." She laughs out loud and smiles as she says "my friends all say that my car smells like smoke, but I don't smell anything. I think they are crazy." She continues to tell me that she loves chocolate and coffee. In fact, she drinks at least six cups of coffee a day and admittedly will put chocolate on anything she can find. When I ask her (with a knowing smile) if she puts chocolate syrup on chocolate bars, her voice gets more confident and louder, "Of course I do!"

Upon examining her, she shows some signs of swelling in her feet. When I asked her about it she says, "it's probably because I eat a lot of potato chips!" and she winks at me. Sally has no co-morbidities. That means at 85 years old she takes no medication, her blood pressure is excellent, her blood sugar is great, and there is no sign of heart disease or cancer. Despite her lifestyle of cigarettes, coffee, chocolate and chips, she'll probably live to be a hundred!

Aubrey, on the other hand is another patient of mine. She is a 22-year-old graduate student. She trains for triathlons, eats a gluten-free and vegan diet and practices yoga. She is a strong proponent for all-natural, whole-food diets and will not let anything artificial, processed, refined or sugary (in other words, delicious!) pass her lips. And when she has children, they most certainly will not eat artificial dyes, candy, gluten, eggs, dairy, or non-vegan cookies and cakes. She makes her own soaps, wears cruelty-free makeup, and only shops from local farmer's markets and organic food stores.

Most of us fall somewhere between Sally and Aubrey. Though I'm sure we'd all love Sally's apparent ability to eat whatever she wants and not gain an ounce!

If you are reading this book, my guess is that you are dissatisfied with something about yourself. Perhaps it is your weight or some other part of your appearance. Maybe you just don't feel good. It could be that you battle mood swings, tiredness, aches, constant hunger and tummy that is always "off."

I've been there. In fact, I still wrestle with many of those areas. But I've also found victory in many of them. And over the years, I've spoken with other women who've struggled and overcome.

This book was written to give you hope. You are not alone in your battle. Though we live in a fallen world and have bodies that are far from perfect, God lavishes His grace on us.

Always remember that our bodies are fearfully and wonderfully made, intricately designed and lovingly handcrafted by the Creator. The world we live in was brought into existence through the unmatched creativity and power of the King of Kings.

So, if we were lovingly created, and our world was a labor of love – then why do we struggle? Why is there a battle within our bodies? Why is there a war raging in our minds and hearts over what we eat and how we take care of our bodies?

The answer may surprise you.

CHAPTER 2

The Price We Pay

...for all have sinned and fall short of the glory of God...

- Romans 3:23

Why do we struggle? If we were so lovingly created, why don't we have perfect bodies?

Actually, we did, but then sin entered God's perfect creation. It infected and tainted everything, including our heart. The beautiful garden grew thorns. Our innocent hearts became rebellious, growing thorns of another kind.

When sin entered the scene, nothing was left unaffected.

What was designed to be a blessing and a gift has become a source of anxiety and bondage. Food went from something that we consumed to something that consumes us. But it doesn't have to be that way.

Just as sin was forever dealt with on the cross, so too have our captive hearts been set free. No longer are we slaves to what we eat.

Jesus replied, "I tell you the truth, everyone who sins is a slave of sin. A slave is not a permanent member of the family, but a son is part of the family forever. So if the Son sets you free, you are truly free.

– John 8:34-36 (NLT)

We've been set free! So why do we still struggle?

The apostle Paul answers that question for us in the letter he wrote to the Philippians.

> *For I have told you often before, and I say it again with tears in my eyes, that there are many whose conduct shows they are really enemies of the cross of Christ. They are headed for destruction.* ***Their god is their appetite****, they brag about shameful things, and they think only about this life here on earth.*
>
> *- Philippians 3:18-19 (NLT, emphasis added)*

You have probably heard it said that the things we give the most time, effort and attention to are what we serve. Those things become our god. And we can easily make our appetite our god, just like the Philippians were doing. And our appetite can be for more than just food, can't it?

The Bible tells us that sin can be grouped into three categories: the desires of the flesh, the lust of the eyes, and the pride of life. All three are related, and all three are deadly.

> *Do not love this world nor the things it offers you, for when you love the world, you do not have the love of the Father in you. For the world offers only* ***a craving for physical pleasure, a craving for everything we see, and pride in our achievements and possessions****. These are not from the Father, but are from this world. And this world is fading away, along with everything that people crave. But anyone who does what pleases God will live forever.*
>
> *– 1 John 2:15-17 (NLT, emphasis added)*

You see, sin is simply desiring something else in place of God.

We turn to food for comfort instead of turning to the Comforter.

We lust after someone we find attractive instead of turning our gaze on the beauty of the Lord.

We become prideful in our accomplishments instead of boasting in what the Lord has done in our lives.

To win the battle for our heart and mind, we can't focus on diminishing our desires for unhealthy things. Instead, we must focus on increasing our desire for our Savior.

> *He must increase, but I must decrease.*
>
> *– John 3:30*

This is an important point, in fact, it is the crux of this whole book - so let's dwell on it for a minute.

If we only battled our negative desires, we'd be facing a never ending (and exhausting!) fight. Due to our fallen sin nature, we would no sooner overcome one unhealthy desire, then to have it replaced by another.

It reminds me of the old joke about the doctor who prescribed aspirin for a patient complaining of a headache. Upon hearing the prescribed remedy, the patient asked the doctor, "Should I also stop banging my head against the wall?"

The doctor had failed to address the underlying cause of the headache. We would make the same mistake if we only addressed our unhealthy desires.

Like Peter attempting to walk on water and getting distracted by the waves, we would fight a losing battle. Only by taking his eyes off the waves and setting them on Jesus was Peter able to make it back into the boat. It is the same for us.

We must recognize that having desires is simply part of our human nature. We must direct these desires toward God. We must look to Him to fulfill our needs. Only then can we experience victory over our negative cravings.

You probably feel like you are stuck in a vicious cycle. I know, I've been there. We get caught in a downward spiral of eating to soothe our stress, only to become stressed by what we are eating.

Thankfully, there is a way out. I will share how you can overcome your desires, how you can turn away from temptation, and how you can walk free.

First, we need to have a better understanding of the connection between what we eat and how we feel, the connection between our mood and our food.

CHAPTER 3

Understanding Emotional Eating

It's been a long day at work.
I've been on my feet since 7:30 AM seeing patient after patient.
Either it's me or something is in the air, because a lot of my patients seem extra emotional, extra sensitive and extra needy today.
I haven't had lunch yet and it's 2:00 PM.
With a 15-minute break, I plop down at the front reception desk next to my friend and co-worker.
I lean my head back and look at her.
She looks at me.
Then she silently reaches under the desk and pulls out a bag of peanut M&Ms.
She slides them over to me without a word.
I smile and take a handful.
She "gets" me.

What is emotional eating? It is an emotional attachment to food in response to stress, and reinforced by the addictive nature of our food today.

This is not a classic eating disorder and it isn't exclusive to young women. A vast number of women in their 30's, 40's and early 50's now find themselves coping with midlife stress by emotional eating. They develop unhealthy lifestyle patterns such as binge eating, yo-yo dieting, calorie restriction and compulsive exercise. While a woman at this age may not consider herself anorexic because she eats regularly, her obsession with maintaining control of food intake or her focus on appearance can be just as destructive.

What is common among emotional eaters is how we have learned to respond to stress and what our bodies have become addicted to. However, it is not completely our fault! (I'll tell you why in the next chapter.)

To help understand the link between stress and eating, we are going to look at two neurohormones that have a huge impact on our stress levels and how we respond to stress.

You are no doubt familiar with the first neurohormone: adrenaline.

Adrenaline gives us the "fight or flight" rush of energy when we are under stress. The release of adrenaline into our bloodstream causes several things to all happen at once:

- It causes an increase in blood flow and oxygen to the brain and muscles
- Our pupils dilate for better vision
- Our heart rate and pulse increase
- Sugar is quickly broken down and released into the bloodstream for instant energy

During fight or flight, our body also shuts down our digestive track and our reproductive and immune systems. Why? Simply put, you don't need any of those systems to run away from a bear, so your body shuts them off to conserve energy and resources.

The second neurohormone produced when we are under stress is cortisol.

Think of adrenaline as lighter fluid and cortisol as charcoal. The lighter fluid (adrenaline) quickly gets the fire going, but it is the charcoal (cortisol) that provides the sustaining fuel for the fire.

Cortisol continues pumping more sugar into your bloodstream so that you have energy to burn. It also meticulously maintains several important body functions:

- Cell repair
- Metabolism (how we break down foods and maintain our energy levels)
- Circadian rhythm (cycles of eating, sleeping, working, etc.)

When expressed appropriately, cortisol is good. When the stressor is gone (e.g., the bear isn't chasing us anymore), our body naturally decreases and maintains a healthy cortisol balance.

When our body is relaxed and stress is not forcing our bodies to make cortisol in response to a "fight or flight" reaction, it can make DHEA. DHEA helps make numerous hormones in our body so that we can optimally break down and use our food, feel good, and sleep well. DHEA is even known as the "anti-aging" hormone.

DHEA is like water thrown on our charcoal; it puts out the cortisol flame after the stressor is gone and negates the potentially bad effects of stress.

However, under periods of long-term stress, we force our bodies to make cortisol continually. This demand means sugar is always available, we are always in "fight or flight" state and our heart is continually working harder. We can't keep up this state forever; our bodies eventually get exhausted.

Imagine trying to put out a forest fire with a water pistol. That is what DHEA is up against when it is trying to regulate cortisol in a continual stress filled existence. No matter how much DHEA you manage to squirt on the fire, the raging cortisol continues to burn at an unrelenting pace. Your body gets exhausted and eventually gives up!

As you might suspect, an abnormal cortisol and DHEA ratio in the body can lead to serious stress-related ailments, such as:

- impairment of the digestive and immune systems
- decreased learning and memory
- increased weight gain (all that sugar floating around your blood stream must be deposited somewhere!)
- fatigue
- increased risk of chronic disease

The bottom line is that we have an out of control fire raging in our bodies and our dinky little DHEA squirt gun is not going to put it out. The longer a fire burns out of control, the more damage is caused.

It boils down to a pretty basic formula:

long term stress + unhealthy food choices
= weight gain and disease

The worst thing we can do is throw more fuel on the fire, and yet that is exactly what happens when we consume carbs, fatty foods and sweets.

"It's not fair!" you exclaim. "Those are exactly the foods I want to eat when I am stressed!"

I know. Me too. But as I mentioned at the end of the last chapter, desiring these foods isn't completely our fault.

There's a good reason our body craves them: there are other neurohormones at work. In the next chapter, we'll look at the neurohormones serotonin and dopamine.

CHAPTER 4

Stress and Serotonin

For several years now I've been counseling Jane for weight loss. She's aware of what healthy eating is and truly enjoys eating well. However, she continues to struggle with the addictive nature of food, especially when she is stressed.

Over the past year, I have watched Jane care for her elderly father whose health is failing. As her father's time on this earth drew closer to an end, I witnessed an emotional change in Jane. Along with a moodier disposition and increased pain levels, she started to eat more as well. And the weight gain was noticeable.

Every few months when I would see her, she had put on more pounds. Finally, at one visit she sat crying in my office and simply said "I am so tired of being this heavy, it's time for a change."

Until that point, Jane was not ready to talk about how food affected her. However, she finally came to a point where she was willing to admit and address her addiction and reliance on food to momentarily mask the pain of watching her father go through a terminal illness.

Can you relate? Food is so much more than a combination of carbs, protein and fat. It has a bigger impact on our bodies than just providing the fuel we need to live. Which is why we need to understand how our body responds to the foods we put in it.

One of the main reasons we choose sweet and carb-heavy foods when we are stressed is due to serotonin.

Serotonin is a neurohormone that is found in the brain, gut and blood cells. Its main role is to promote the feeling of satisfaction and may also help to regulate mood and sleep. Altered serotonin levels can lead to mood disturbances, fatigue and gut issues (such as irritable bowel syndrome).

The Lord has designed our bodies to be able to make serotonin through exercise, exposure to bright light, and through our diet. We can make serotonin with the amino acid tryptophan (high in turkey, milk, lentils, beans, nuts, and oats), vitamin B6 and magnesium.

> *Anyone who celebrates Thanksgiving with a traditional turkey dinner has certainly felt the full effects of serotonin. Not only does turkey contain high levels of tryptophan (a precursor to serotonin), but eating complex carbs like mashed potatoes, sweet potato casserole, and stuffing also produce serotonin. To top it off, sweet treats are another serotonin trigger. So all those post-turkey dinner desserts add even more serotonin to the mix. No wonder everyone needs a nap after Thanksgiving dinner!*

We feel better when we eat these foods because they raise our hormone production, but it is only temporary.

As with any substance that increases our pleasure and makes us feel good (even temporarily), it can be habit forming.

If we reach for sweet or fatty foods whenever stress comes knocking, it can quickly become an unconscious habit. Soon we'll find ourselves automatically seeking out these comfort foods whenever our stress levels start to rise.

We begin to find ourselves doing it without even realizing! That is the power of reinforced bad habits. We can become ignorant of our level of bondage to them - until we try to break them that is. At that point, it becomes clear how entrenched these habits are in our lives – and how much work it will take to break free of them.

The trick is that we can't just try to eliminate these bad habits – we must replace them with good habits and healthy responses to stress.

Imagine a tall glass of water. But instead of clean drinking water, the glass is full of filthy sludge. Our imaginary glass of water can't be tipped over and spilled out. The only way to change the contents of the glass is to pour more water in to displace the old water.

Obviously, pouring more dirty water in won't help our situation. The only solution is to pour crystal clear water in. At first, it won't seem like much is happening. The dirty sludge water still contaminates the glass. But slowly, little by little, the dirty water is displaced – going from black sludge to brownish, to cloudy and finally to crystal clear.

The same goes for getting rid of improper desires. Deleting desires isn't the answer, replacing negative desires with positive ones is the only long-term solution.

The apostle Paul gave the same advice to the church in Rome:

> *And so, dear brothers and sisters, I plead with you to give your bodies to God because of all he has done for you. Let them be a living and holy sacrifice—the kind he will find acceptable. This is truly the way to worship him. Don't copy the behavior and customs of this world, but let God transform you into a new person by changing the way you think. Then you will learn to know God's will for you, which is good and pleasing and perfect.*
>
> *– Romans 12:1-2 (NLT, emphasis added)*

Women's magazines are constantly touting headlines that promise easy ways to transform your body. Paul says the first and most important step it to let God transform our mind.

When we submit our lives to the Lord, He will pour into us His Holy Spirit, and if we continue to submit and obey, our old habits and fleshly desires will be displaced. Soon enough we will find that we are full of joy in the Lord, celebrating the freedom we have through His Son. Once our minds are transformed, our bodies will begin to follow suit.

In the next chapter, we'll look at one last neurohormone that comes into play when we are under stress.

CHAPTER 5

The Dopamine Dilemma

I have a friend who has a problem. She will come home from a stressful day at work, eat a big dinner and then open a bag of chips. Before she even realizes it, the entire bag is gone. She admits that she is not even hungry while she eats the chips. Many times, she is not aware of how much she has eaten until she reaches for another chip, only to have her hand hit the empty bottom of the bag. What drives this kind of behavior? Dopamine.

Dopamine is a "feel good" neurotransmitter and is found in concentrated levels in the pleasure centers of the brain. A deficiency in this neurohormone can lead to depression, dissatisfaction, cravings and addictions.

Foods that trigger our dopamine receptors include simple carbs (sugar), alcohol, coffee, vegetable oils and diet soda. We all recognize that these foods are potentially addictive, and dopamine is the reason why!

Sugar is very dopamine stimulating. A high level of sugar in our diet causes our body to respond by "down regulating" our dopamine receptors (decreasing the number of receptors which reduces our sensitivity).

When we consume sugar, dopamine is released and gives us a "feel good" feeling. However, the next time we eat sugar, the effect is blunted. So, we need to eat more and more sugar to get the same effects of satisfaction and pleasure.

Talk about a vicious cycle!

For example, are you familiar with Dove chocolate squares? You know those little one inch by one inch packets of deliciousness that are so easy to pop in your mouth?

My friend Elizabeth loves Dove chocolates. She especially loves them at work. She told me the other day that she started to track her diet using a new phone app and noticed something. She used to be able to eat only one piece of chocolate and feel satisfied. Now, as she works longer hours and deals with increased stress due to an upcoming move, she found herself eating three pieces of chocolate.

She wasn't even aware that she increased her portion size by two pieces… she just ate until she was satisfied. She realized that the satisfaction she received from sugary foods was being blunted and now she needs more food (or sugar) to have that same amount of stress-relief satisfaction.

But once again, there is hope! Instead of eating junk food we can make our own dopamine by consuming the right foods.

Foods high in tyrosine (the building block of dopamine) include chicken, ricotta cheese, oatmeal, dark chocolate, wheat germ and fava beans.

We can also make dopamine through touch (hugs), massage, intimacy, and laughter.

At this point, you may be having an "Aha!" moment. "That explains why I absolutely love and crave chocolate chip cookies after a long day at work!"

Here's my personal "fail-proof stress cure" recipe:

- A dash of dark chocolate
- 2 heaping measures of hugs from my girls
- Mix in a humorous exchange of texts with a friend
- Top off with a generous dollop of snuggle time with my husband

Consuming this potent combination never fails to melt my stress away!

Over the last few chapters we've looked at four neurohormones and the role they play in our bodies when stress is introduced. Hopefully you have a better understanding of how your body responds, and perhaps how not to respond to stress.

But maybe you are still not sure if you are emotionally connected to the food you eat. The short quiz in the next chapter will answer that question once and for all.

CHAPTER 6

Quiz: Am I An Emotional Eater?

1. Do you frequently eat when you feel emotional but not particularly hungry?

When a craving comes from an emotion or something other than hunger, eating cannot satisfy it. If you are eating but don't physically need the food, you'll never feel satisfied. In fact, research has found that dieters who eat according to internal emotional cues, such as loneliness or boredom, instead of physical cues, have hindered weight loss attempts and poor weight management.

2. Instead of confronting a problem, do you head to the refrigerator?

Your kids aren't obeying. You just had a disagreement with your husband. The house is a mess. You're overwhelmed. Suddenly the only thing you can think about is eating something.

Psychologists say that numbing yourself with food rather than dealing with your feelings can increase stress, which in turn can raise your blood pressure and weaken your immune system. This in turn can lead to further emotional eating. It's a vicious cycle!

3. Do you "punish" yourself after eating a treat?

Guilt can lead to uncontrolled eating. For example, you are handed a large piece of cake at a birthday party. Instead of enjoying the cake and eating until you are satisfied, you continually think about the calories, sugar and "bad fats" in the icing with each bite. Now you've destroyed any pleasure you had hoped to derive from that cake. Instead of eating until you are satisfied (which may only be half of that piece of cake) you eat the entire piece of cake begrudgingly.

Or, do you eat that whole piece of birthday cake while promising yourself to make sure you exercise "extra hard" the next day to make up for it? While adjusting exercise to account for caloric intake can be a good idea at times, a strenuous exercise routine to "punish" ourselves for eating something indulgent is harmful.

4. Do you regularly overeat carb heavy, fatty or sweet foods?

You know—the ones you crave the most. Do you eat until you can't eat any more? Do you still eat even though you know you've had enough? Like my friend in the previous chapter, do you eat a whole bag of something without even realizing it?

Summary

Don't worry, I won't ask you how you scored. My guess is that you answered "yes" to at least one of the questions above, maybe even several.

The simple fact is, if you are a woman, you are prone to emotional eating (no, that is not a stereotype; it is simply the way we are wired!).

Emotional eating often has undiagnosed but three very real physical underpinnings:

- Stress
- Hormonal and neurotransmitter imbalances
- Food sensitivities

We'll take a deeper look at these three emotional eating catalysts in the next chapter.

Craving Catalysts

I had a particularly stressful event happen at work the other day. As soon as I got home, I went straight to my stash of dark chocolate, only to be horrified by what I saw! My husband walked in to find me on the floor in tears. There was no dark chocolate anywhere in the house! Like a knight in shining armor, he quickly ran to the store and brought back what I craved most in the world at that moment. You might think I downed the entire bar in one sitting, but I only ate a single square. That was all I needed to soothe the overwhelming craving I had for dark chocolate at that moment.

Why do we have these kinds of uncontrollable cravings for chocolate or potato chips? There are likely a multitude of factors that play into our cravings, but there are three triggers that are specially to blame: stress, hormonal imbalances and food sensitivities. Let's take a look at each.

Stress

We are women and we carry the weight and responsibility of our households, our husbands, children, parents, occupations... you name it. There are tons of opportunities for stress and sometimes life just "gets to us."

Stress is a likely the number one catalyst that drives uncontrollable cravings. Even if you don't feel stressed out or you consider yourself to be a laid-back person, stress plays a bigger role in your cravings than you may realize. We've covered stress quite a bit in the last few chapters and I'm going to dig more into it in a later chapter. Therefore, let's move on to the next catalyst.

Hormonal and Neurotransmitter Imbalances

Hormonal and neurotransmitter imbalances can spark insatiable cravings that contribute to overeating. I've had good success in treating patients with targeted support in the form of amino acids (adequate protein intake), vitamins and mineral cofactors.

We need the necessary nutritional building blocks for our bodies to function at the optimal level. These building blocks do not come from processed, fatty and sugary foods. They are ideally found in whole foods, the ones that were naturally designed by our Creator.

One major building block (and a common deficiency in women) is protein. Protein supplies necessary amino acids such as tryptophan and tyrosine which support our endocrine system, boost our metabolism, and create our "feel good" and "sleep good" hormones.

At a minimum, the recommended daily intake of protein is 0.8 grams of protein for every kilogram of body weight, but ideally we want to aim for 1.2 grams of protein for every kilogram of body weight.

Want some help with the math? Take your weight in pounds and divide by 2.2 to get your weight in kilograms. Then multiply that number by 0.8 to get a minimum amount of protein (in grams) that you need to eat in a day. Multiply it by 1.2 to get the goal (in grams) you should shoot for each day.

Let's look at an example of a woman who weighs 150 pounds. First divide 150 by 2.2, which equals 68 (her weight in kilograms). Now multiple 68 by 0.8 (the minimum recommended daily intake), which equals 54. That is her minimum number of grams of protein she should be consuming each day.

If she ate two eggs, one cup of cooked chicken breast and a cheese stick every day, she would eat at least 54 grams of protein. Doesn't seem like much, does it? It's not really, and it's not usually enough for women to stay energized and satisfied. That's why I recommend aiming for 1.2 grams of protein per kilogram of body weight per day.

Let's look back at our example woman. Take her 68 kilograms of bodyweight and multiply it by 1.2 (our goal intake), which equals 81. Sounds like a lot more, doesn't it? Well, not necessarily.

Here's how you could easily reach this amount: breakfast would be two eggs, mid-morning snack would be a cheese stick, lunch would be one half cup of chicken on a salad with a handful of almonds, a midafternoon snack would be half of a cup of Greek yogurt and dinner would be a chicken breast, a half cup of quinoa and veggies. That would give you well over 85 grams of protein!

Now, having all this protein is excellent for you, but what good is that protein if you do not have any other essential building blocks for your hormones? You will need adequate B vitamins (namely Vitamin B6), Vitamin C and minerals like zinc and magnesium to take those amino acids and make them into your hormones.

When working with patients, I will typically supplement these vitamins and minerals with the long-term goal that my patients will eventually be able to eat these vitamins in their diet. However, most people have underlying health conditions or are undergoing significant amounts of stress that make a supplementation regime a smart choice. This is especially the case with magnesium.

> *Magnesium is a mineral that is used for over 300 reactions in your body. It supports your nervous, muscular, skeletal, endocrine (hormone), and cardiovascular systems. It is a relaxing supplement and a vasodilator (meaning that it helps to decrease blood pressure). It also helps increase bowel movements. Many people will see noticeable positive changes by just adding this supplement without any other dietary adjustments.*

Do you have a suspicion that you need magnesium? Although this is not totally diagnostic, I usually ask my patients a few questions that helps me decide if we should supplement with magnesium. One question is "do you prefer chocolate over vanilla?" or "do you crave chocolate during that certain time of the month?" If the answer is an emphatic "Yes!" then they could probably benefit from magnesium supplementation. You see, the Lord has designed us to naturally desire foods that are beneficial for us (in moderation). We crave foods that are high in nutrient value, including the vitamins and minerals we need.

Want to guess what food is high in magnesium? Yep, chocolate! Dark chocolate (having 70% cocoa or more) contains about 145 mg of magnesium in every 100 ounces (half of a chocolate bar). That is almost half of the recommended daily allowance of magnesium for women. When we are cranky and crampy (especially around the start of our cycles), we tend to gravitate towards foods that will relax us, increase blood flow, and decrease spasm and cramps. Since chocolate is that amazing combination of sugar and magnesium, our brain tells us to "eat up!"

But as we have seen, the sugary content of some chocolates can be addictive and not beneficial in large amounts. So why not supplement with magnesium? I could almost guarantee that you will crave less chocolate when you supplement with magnesium.

I have one patient who was a chocolate addict. We started her on a magnesium supplementation and within two weeks she excitedly told me that she no longer craved chocolate. She still ate it and enjoyed it, but it no longer had the power over her as before, she no longer felt that she "needed" to eat it.

Is your craving for sugary treats (not necessarily chocolate)? Then you may be deficient in vitamin C. Vitamin C is classically known to be the "immune system" vitamin. However, Vitamin C does a lot more. It helps to maintain integrity of cells, supports collagen and vasculature, supports hormone production and metabolic function. It is imperative we have enough of this vitamin!

Most animals can make vitamin C. However, the Lord designed a few animals, in addition to humans, not to be able to make vitamin C. If we cannot make this essential vitamin, then we must eat it. Most vitamin C foods have a sweeter quality to them (think oranges, sweet bell peppers, kiwi, strawberries, etc.). Therefore, a strong craving for sweets may mean that you need more vitamin C foods in your diet or even supplementation.

However, not all supplements are appropriate for every person, and as with any healthcare intervention, there are possible risks. So, talk to your doctor today about what vitamin and mineral supplementation is right for you. (Yeah, I know - I sound like a TV commercial!)

Food Sensitivities

Food sensitivities can also be a major source of food addiction and emotional eating. We crave the foods we are sensitive to because we've grown used to the abnormal biochemical state those foods produce in our body.

It sounds strange, doesn't it? But more and more research is showing that we physically become dependent on the foods that are harming us. This dependence is usually intense as well.

For example, I can usually tell which of my patients are potentially sensitive to gluten (the protein found in wheat, barley and rye) when they reveal their dependence on carb-heavy foods. I had a patient tell me one time "I would rather that you shoot me in the face than take away my bread." Wow, what a statement! And what a red flag for a potential food dependency. If a patient makes a statement like this, it is usually a result of a strong dependency on the hormones that bread makes in their body (serotonin and dopamine) or a food sensitivity.

Up next is a simple test that you can do on your own that may reveal if you have a food sensitivity.

CHAPTER 8

The Tongue Test

D
o you suspect that you may have an undiagnosed food
sensitivity? It is becoming more and more common in our
culture today. You can see your doctor to get tested for
allergies and sensitivities, but you can also try a simple "tongue
test." I'll go over the process of administrating a tongue test on
yourself, but first, it is important to understand a bit more about food
sensitivities.

Our gut is known as the "second brain." It has millions of
neurons and neurohormones functioning every day. There truly is a
"gut feeling" which is innate and reflexive, and it is a result of
hormones made in the gut.

Serotonin is one hormone potentially produced in response to a
food sensitivity. If there is an imbalance of this hormone, we may
experience altered bowel movements and intestinal problems.

However, you don't need a lab test to find out whether you have
a food sensitivity. An elimination diet can help you to identify
potential problem foods.

*An elimination diet removes highly allergenic foods from your diet for
at least 21 days. Foods that are considered highly allergenic include:*

dairy, gluten, soy, citrus, tomatoes, eggs, corn and peanuts. Removal of these foods gives the intestinal tract and body time to heal and be nourished while you eat minimally processed, whole and hypoallergenic foods.

Symptoms such as fatigue, stomach problems, headaches, rashes, or even menstrual problems may become much better during the elimination diet. After 21 days, the allergenic foods are slowly added back in, one food at time, one week at a time. Upon reintroducing the allergenic foods, you will have a good idea if you have a food sensitivity if those previous symptoms return or get worse.

An alternative to an elimination diet is the Neuro Lingual Coca stress test. The immunologist that developed this test back in the 1950s found that if you ingest a food that you are allergic or sensitive to, your body will make stress hormones. The response of your body to foods is almost immediate because of the connection between the nerves in your tongue to your cranial nerves and brain.

If you recall, our body releases adrenaline when we are under stress, which increases your pulse rate. So, the premise behind this test is that if you eat a food you are sensitive to, you will register a stress response and immediately your pulse will increase.

Want to try it out? It is an easy test to administer to yourself at home, and possibly a quick way to identify potential food sensitivities.

To start the test, sit down in a quiet spot and rest for at least 5 minutes. After 5 minutes, take your resting heart rate. Using the pulse at your neck or wrist, count your heartbeats for a full 60 seconds. Now eat a bite of food that you suspect you are sensitive to. Chew it well, savor the flavor and swallow. Take your pulse again (for a full 60 seconds) and see if there is any change. If you have a food sensitivity, your pulse rate may be higher during this second test.

Keep in mind that your body may naturally increase your heart rate upon eating anything, so we are looking for an elevation in heart rate of 6 beats or more.

I recently spoke at a ladies Health and Wellness Day at my church. During my presentation, I had the ladies perform this test with a piece of Matzo bread. It is a good food to test for gluten sensitivity since it is made from just wheat flour and water (it is always better to test with a simple food since more complex foods - like a cupcake - have multiple ingredients and you won't know which one your body is reacting to).

After performing the test, about 8 women out of the forty that were present, found that their pulses had increased. Two of those women had known gluten (wheat) sensitivities. Another woman has a daughter who has a gluten sensitivity but she had not considered herself to be sensitive prior to the test.

There was also a young woman who tested positive and who was just starting an elimination diet because she suspected that she had a food sensitivity. She told me a few weeks later that after completing the elimination diet, she found that she had strong reactions when she reintroduced gluten. She said to me "every time I eat it, I get terrible stomach aches now. I guess that tongue test was right!"

I encourage you to try it, even if you don't think you are sensitive to any foods. You may be surprised to discover that a food sensitivity is at the root of seemingly unrelated symptoms.

Keep in mind that this test is not foolproof. It is not considered a truly diagnostic test for food sensitivities. If you believe you may have a food sensitivity, try an elimination diet or speak to a nutritionist.

In the last few chapters, we've covered many of the physical sources of stress and how our body responds. Next, we'll look at the emotional and spiritual side of things.

CHAPTER 9

Sources of Stress

Hopefully you now have a good grasp on how our hormones and external factors can lead to emotional eating. Next, let's turn our attention to the spiritual and emotional response to food. What is the source of our stress and is it causing us to eat things we shouldn't?

We Don't Feel Worthy

Are you tired of trying to keep up with the world's expectations? Expectations of how we should look, act, and speak? What about trying to keep up with our perceived expectations at church?

Relax. Take a deep breath.

Romans 8:16 says that we are God's children. We belong to Him.

Below is a short list of statements from the Bible that are true about you if you are a child of God and Jesus Christ is your Lord and Savior. These statements aren't true about you someday. They aren't only for the super-sanctified or the passionately-pious. They are true about you at the very instant you commit your life to Christ.

Bonus: for the full list, turn to Appendix 1

Read through the list slowly. If there is a statement that you find hard to believe, look up the Bible verse and read it for yourself. I encourage you to read through the list often. I know some women who read it daily and have found it life changing!

> **<u>I am accepted…</u>**
>
> *I am God's child. - John 1:12*
>
> *I have been justified. - Romans 5:1*
>
> *I am complete in Christ. - Colossians 2:9-10*
>
> **<u>I am secure…</u>**
>
> *I am free from condemnation. - Romans 8:1-2*
>
> *I am a citizen of heaven. - Philippians 3:20*
>
> *I have not been given a spirit of fear but of power, love and a sound mind. - 2 Timothy 1:7*
>
> **<u>I am significant…</u>**
>
> *I am God's temple. - 1 Corinthians 3:16*
>
> *I am God's workmanship. - Ephesians 2:10*
>
> *I can do all things through Christ, who strengthens me. - Philippians 4:13*[1]

We Feel Out of Control

Many of us feel like we need to control our circumstances so that we can achieve the desired outcome. And if we are not in control or it doesn't seem like we are getting what we want, then we worry about our present circumstances. But the Lord says:

Be anxious for nothing, but in everything by prayer and supplication, with thanksgiving, let your requests be made known to God.

– Philippians 4:6-7

Guess what? Our God is the same yesterday, today and forever, His Spirit resides in our hearts and His Son, our Savior, continually makes intercession for us before the Throne of Grace.

Yours, O Lord, is the greatness,
The power and the glory,
The victory and the majesty;
For all that is in heaven and in earth is Yours;
Yours is the kingdom, O Lord,
And You are exalted as head over all.

- I Chronicles 29:11

And the High King of Heaven wants to help you:

My help comes from the Lord, Who made heaven and earth.

- Psalm 121:2

I am going to share more about this in the next chapter, but worry and anxiety have always been a struggle for me. What helped me immensely through my battle was saturating my mind in Scripture. I had a worry journal that I carried around with all my favorite Scripture in it.

Bonus: You'll find my list of "Worry Scripture" in Appendix 2. It has brought me through some tough times and I hope you are blessed by it as well.

We Feel Like We Need to Numb Feelings

Some women cope by silently suffering, learning to soothe and satisfy their feelings with food. We can preoccupy ourselves with food to prevent unwanted feelings - including pain, loneliness, unworthiness, boredom, exhaustion, and shame. We say, "You know what? I just want to feel good for a little bit." And so, we eat.

Maybe you are like me, sometimes reaching the point of feeling a little like ash. We become dried out, easily scattered; like we are just blowing in the wind and going through the motions.

If you can relate, take heart. Jesus is in the business of transforming ashes.

Isaiah 61:1-3 says:

> *"The Spirit of the Lord God is upon Me, because the Lord has anointed Me*
> *To preach good tidings to the poor;*
> *He has sent Me to heal the brokenhearted,*
> *To proclaim liberty to the captives,*
> *And the opening of the prison to those who are bound;*
> *To proclaim the acceptable year of the Lord,*
> *And the day of vengeance of our God;*
> *To comfort all who mourn,*
> *To console those who mourn in Zion,*
> *To give them beauty for ashes,*
> *The oil of joy for mourning,*
> *The garment of praise for the spirit of heaviness;*
> *That they may be called trees of righteousness,*
> *The planting of the Lord, that He may be glorified."*

The Lord does amazing things, transforming and conforming us for our good and for His glory when we surrender our ashes to Him!

We Long for Companionship

There is nothing wrong with desiring fellowship - a cup of coffee and laughter with our friends on a Saturday afternoon is a wonderful thing. In fact, coffee with a friend is a great way to get the dopamine flowing, especially if chocolate is also involved!

However, we need to be wary of food becoming the focal point of our gatherings. In our culture today, we use food as an excuse to get together. And to add insult to injury, the clear majority of our favorite "celebration" foods are fat-laden and calorie-dense.

For example, one glass of soda is typically 180 calories and would require walking at a moderate pace for 40 minutes to burn off. How about just 10 potato chips with 1 tablespoon of ranch dip? Doesn't seem like much, right? Well, you would have to bike 20 minutes to burn off those calories. Dare I talk about cheesecake? For one small slice of cheesecake, you would have to either walk for 75 minutes, bike for 35 minutes, swim for 35 minutes, or run for 30 minutes to burn off the average 285 calories that it contains.

Thankfully, there are plenty of wonderful food choices that we can substitute for these common belly-busters. A little extra planning and preparation can go a long way in still delivering a fun get together while also protecting ourselves and our families from consuming a day's worth of calories in the span of a few hours.

Bonus: See Appendix 3 for a list of great websites and resources for healthy recipes and snack ideas.

We eat because we feel insignificant or unworthy. We eat to cope with feelings of life being out of our control and moving in directions we don't want. We eat to numb feelings and alleviate anxiety. And we eat because it is what we do when we get together with friends and family.

The next step to overcoming our poor habits of emotional eating is to recognize when we eat and how we feel at that time - because they are directly linked. We'll explore more of this in the next chapter.

CHAPTER 10

Recognize Your Emotions

Y ou've probably heard of a prayer journal before. And perhaps you keep a personal journal. But have you heard of a food journal? It goes something like this:

Dear Food Journal,

I love iced coffee. I can't get enough. Dunkin' Donuts, Tim Hortons, McDonalds - it doesn't matter to me, I love them all. If it is cold and creamy and maybe with a fun shot of flavor (mmm... cookies and cream!), then I don't care where it comes from.

Do you think six a day is too many? Yeah, I don't either. Thanks for the validation! Come to think of it, it's been almost an hour since my last iced coffee - time to go grab another one. Maybe I should get two? You know, just in case they run out later.

Do you think there will be iced coffee in heaven? Maybe if I get raptured with an iced coffee in my hand I'll be able to bring it to heaven. And maybe it will be like that oil jar in the Bible that never runs dry! I'll have to ask my pastor about that one.

Thanks for the talk, Food Journal! Do you want me to pick up an
iced coffee for you too? My treat! And if you don't finish it, I'd be
happy to help. =)
    Love,
    Erica

OK, so that is not exactly how a food journal goes. And my iced
coffee addiction is not quite as bad as that.

Here's the plan: to discover and identify how close food and
mood are linked, I want you to keep a food journal for a few days.

Here's how it works.

For the next few days, before you eat anything (even a handful
of grapes), I want you to write down what you're feeling and
thinking at that exact moment. Seeing your emotions on paper will
help you understand what's happening inside and will help you
recognize times when you're more likely to eat because of
something other than hunger.

When I counsel patients in the clinic, I will ask them to record
food and emotions for three days. Patients are usually surprised by
two things: first, how much they eat in a day (or how few good
things like veggies they eat); and second, that the more stressful the
day, the poorer their food choices become.

Remember my friend Elizabeth from chapter five? Until she
started tracking her food, she didn't realize she was eating more
chocolate than she used to.

You also need to note when and where you are eating these
foods. Is it while you are sitting at your desk working? Sitting in
front of the TV or reading? One hour before dinner? Right after an
argument with your husband?

Perhaps you find yourself reaching for a sweet after having a
conversation like this with your five-year old (or maybe it is just
me):

"Abbie put your shoes on please, it is almost time to go.

No, you can't wear a crown to school today, now put your shoes on honey.

Hurry and take one more bite of cereal, and where's your shoes?

Abbie, we are walking out the door... why are your shoes not on?!"

Suddenly there is chocolate in my hand. I have no idea how it got there, it just appeared. And now I need to wash down the chocolate with an iced coffee!

That is where the food journal comes in. When we are forced to record everything that goes in our mouths for a few days, we may be very surprised at the results.

So, to recap, your food journal should have five columns: when, what, amount/size, thoughts/feelings, and circumstances. That way we can record when we are eating (time of day), what we are eating, the serving size (e.g., handful of M&Ms, medium iced coffee, half of a grilled chicken salad), our emotional state while eating (e.g., stressed, angry, tired, worried, upset, happy, bored, etc.), and the circumstances (e.g., ate after meeting with boss, had snack right before big presentation).

For an example of a very simple food diary, please see Appendix 4.

Not a fan of "hard copy" records? There are many good food diary apps for your phone. I personally like to use LiveStrong.com's MyPlate Calorie Tracker app. Although it's bit tougher to record emotional states or circumstances while eating, it's a nice tool to track what and how much we eat throughout the day.

Keep this up for at least three days. Yes, I know it can be tedious. And I know it can be hard to find the time. But the payoff is worth it. I guarantee it will be an eye-opening experience for you.

One way to speed up the process during your day (especially if you are super busy… and who isn't?!) is to use your cell phone to take a quick pic of everything you eat and drink during the day. Then at the end of the day, you can sit down with your food journal and go back through your pics and record the information.

If you find that you are emotionally eating (i.e., you are reaching for food when stressed/upset/etc. instead of eating out of hunger), then we need to deal with it. The trick is to identify your triggers and then replace food as your stress-soother with something else. In our case, the "something else" is the promises and provision of our Savior.

What does this look like? Personally, I keep my favorite scripture close at hand. Whether it is verses I memorized that I repeat to myself, or a list of scriptures (see appendix) that I have printed out and keep strategically within reach (at my desk, in my purse, next to my bed).

For others, it may be prayer. Or you might use worship songs. Put some of your favorite songs on your phone (or pull up Pandora or YouTube) and play a couple of songs when the urge to eat comes. This will help to distract from the immediate impulse of wanting to reach for food, and it will help realign our thoughts and emotions so that we can set our eyes on Jehovah Jireh, our Provider.

Remember our passage about not letting our bellies be our god?

Dear brothers and sisters, pattern your lives after mine, and learn from those who follow our example. For I have told you often before, and I say it again with tears in my eyes, that there are many whose conduct shows they are really enemies of the cross of Christ. They are headed for destruction. Their god is their appetite, they brag about shameful things, and they think only about this life here on earth.

- Philippians 3:17-19 (NLT, emphasis added)

We decide what to put into our bodies all day long. When we make that decision to eat, is our god our bellies? Are we giving in to the craving for that soda or second serving of cookies because we are stressed? Or is our god the King above all heaven and earth who loves us more than we can ever imagine and has a special plan for our lives? We need our bodies to be healthy and fully functional so that we can be used for His purpose. We are not as effective if we are defeated, exhausted, achy and cranky all the time!

> *Therefore, whether you eat or drink, or whatever you do, do all to the glory of God.*
>
> *- I Corinthians 10:31*

My major trigger for emotional eating was anxiety and fear. As I'll share in the next chapter, God did an amazing work in my life to free me from that bondage.

CHAPTER 11

My Story

As we transition into the more practical portion of this book, I want us to consider realistic expectations for ourselves.

The Word of God and our personal walk with Jesus have incredible power to deliver us from the things of this world that consume us and dominate our thoughts and influence our emotions.

We all have battles. Some of us battle with depression. Some of us battle with lusts. Others battle with gossip, vanity or love of possessions. My battle has always been with fear and anxiety.

Since I was a teen, I can remember being self-conscience about who I was (what teen wasn't?) and therefore fearful of what others thought of me. That fear gradually took hold of me and transformed into a fear of many things... including public speaking, flying, confined spaces, heights, and even being in meetings where the door was closed or I didn't have direct access to an exit.

Interestingly enough, I never really experienced intense fear until I was born again. It was not my new relationship with Jesus that caused these fears - it was the fact that I was now an enemy of Satan. The moment I was saved, I became an ambassador for the Kingdom of God. The enemy fights to render us useless in whatever ways he can, to make us ineffective ambassadors. Satan wanted my mind and my actions to disgrace the Lord. God wanted to use my weaknesses to display His strength, to humble my heart and glorify Himself through my life.

The Lord has been so faithful to me and has given me great victories in the area of fear. A few years ago, I was involved in a woman's Bible Study at church that was specifically about breaking the chains of sin and bondage through our relationship with Jesus. During this time, the battle in my mind was intense and the Lord allowed several trials of refinement to come into my life.

One of the biggest trials was traveling for work. At one point, I was required to travel once a month for 4 months down to Raleigh, NC. This involved traveling alone (yikes!) on a plane (double yikes!). I had to get on a plane 16 different times (due to indirect flights) which truly stretched me, to say the least!

To keep my fears in check, I needed to continually remind myself of the sweet truth that even in the midst of trials, God is ultimately in control. Satan asked for permission to test Job and to sift Peter like wheat. In "The Strategy of Satan," Warren Wiersbe says "We can be sure that when Satan turns up the heat in our lives, God controls the thermostat! Job had no idea what was going on behind the scenes. He had no idea that God was permitting him to suffer so that Satan may be silenced. The 'real battle' was 'in the Heavenly places' (Ephesians 6:12)."2

Looking back at my trials, I see God's refinement in me, His glory revealed, and Satan being silenced. As awful as it was sometimes, I would not trade my experience for any amount of comfort. Through those trials, the Lord taught me the real origin of my deception and how to overcome it.

The first trip was especially scary. I had intense fear of the unknown. I had never really traveled alone before and would be responsible for getting on the plane, getting to Raleigh, getting a taxi and getting to the conference all on my own. The enemy was planting terrible thoughts in my mind such as: "You can't do this!", "You are all alone!", and "What makes you think that God will come through for you this time? If you haven't learned your lesson to trust Him by now, you never will!"

The Bible describes Satan as a "roaring lion." He hurls accusations and condemnation at us, hoping that we will respond in fear - that we'll lie down, give up, and lose hope. If we listen to his lies, that's exactly how we'll respond. So how do we withstand the roar?

Submit to God

Therefore submit to God. Resist the devil and he will flee from you.

- James 4:7

I started off this trip telling God exactly how nervous and anxious I was. But through it I learned that I needed to trust Him in all things and love Him no matter the circumstances. Loving God meant...

Thank Him for the Trials

Always give thanks to God the Father for everything, in the name of our Lord Jesus Christ.
- Ephesians 5:20 (NCV)

In everything give thanks; for this is God's will for us in Christ Jesus.
- I Thessalonians 5:18

This didn't mean that I enjoyed my trials. But I thanked God for each opportunity for Him to stretch me and refine me.

Spend Time in the Word

I spent most of my first few trips with my head down, buried in my Bible and my "worry" Scripture journal. The Lord spoke to me and comforted me with passages such as:

> *I know the Lord is always with me. I will not be shaken, for he is right beside me.* - Psalm 16:8 (NLT)
>
> *I will trust in him and not be afraid.* - Isaiah 12:2 (NLT)
>
> *But I am trusting you, O Lord... My future is in your hands.* - Psalm 31:14-15 (NLT)
>
> *Do not worry about anything...* - Philippians 4:6 (NCV)

During my second trip down to North Carolina, I felt confident in the Lord and almost worry free. I felt like the battle was finally over! Then the way back up to New York was one of my darkest times ever. I don't know if it was the enemy hitting me hard because I was feeling confident in the Lord or if it was the next step in the Lord's refinement (or both!), but I hit rock bottom. At 7:00 AM, I stood at the boarding gate and almost did not get on. My hands were sweaty and shaking, I was shivering and my teeth were chattering. I felt light headed and I literally ran back and forth to the ladies' room every 10 minutes for an hour. I felt my heart ache as I tried to imagine myself on that plane. It was a full-blown panic attack! And I knew that if I didn't get on that plane, I wouldn't make it home to my family.

As I boarded, I buried my nose in Romans chapter 8. I must have read the whole chapter 3 times before take-off. It brought me just enough comfort to keep me from vomiting and running off the plane screaming like a mad woman! I kept returning to verses 14 and 15:

For all who are led by the Spirit of God are children of God. So, you have not received a spirit that makes you fearful slaves. Instead, you received God's Spirit when he adopted you as his own children. Now we call him, "Abba, Father."

I remember looking out the window as we taxied out and seeing a dark, rainy, cold day. Everything was so gray and I felt so hopeless. Why couldn't I just kick this habit of fear? Why does it always seem to come back? I felt my spirit trying hard to "get a grip."

As the plane took off and we climbed higher and higher, I almost lost control. Then suddenly (as if on cue), the plane broke through the dark clouds and I saw nothing but pure blue light. Above the storm was a clear sky full of beautiful big clouds, sunshine and the most amazing color blue I have ever seen.

It was a perfect moment and I remember feeling as if the Lord was giving me a very special treasure. That treasure was for me and me alone. I envisioned the Lord's strong and mighty hand holding up that plane, guiding it towards the beautiful heavens... just like He's always held me up and guided me through all the storms towards His blessings. When I finally looked away from that marvelous site, my eyes fell to the words of Romans 8:35...

Who shall separate us from the love of Christ?...

In a wonderful daze of Spirit filled peace, I made it home safely. On the ride home from the Syracuse airport, I heard a sermon on the local Christian radio station. Something the teacher said really struck: "when we fear circumstances and people, our focus cannot be on God. And because of that, we are unable to accomplish what the Lord has called us to do. It's like He has this incredible, magnificent story that He is weaving and He's invited us to take a part in His Story. This life is not about me... it's all about Him." I realized in that moment that there was a fourth step in battling the Enemy.

This fourth step is so important, it gets its own chapter.

CHAPTER 12

Trials Bring God the Glory

In the last chapter, we covered three ways to battle the enemy in the midst of a trial: submit to God, thank Him for the trials, and spend lots of time in the Word and learn His character. The fourth way to battle the enemy in the midst of a trial is to *look for ways to glorify Christ*.

What does that look like? Before I share my personal example, let me share a story from one of my favorite authors. In his book, It's Not About Me, Pastor Max Lucado shares a story about a friend of his who is fighting cancer. The cancer was ravaging not only the man's body, but also his faith. It seemed his prayers for healing were not being answered and he wondered if it was due to a weak faith. Lucado suggested a different answer. "It's not about you," he told his friend. "Your hospital room is a showcase for your Maker."

What did Lucado mean? He meant that his friend had a unique opportunity to exhibit hope and joy to those around him, despite his pain and heartache. When Lucado saw his friend again, he noted a significant change. His friend now saw his sickness in the light of God's sovereign plan for his life. He became a missionary to the cancer ward. "I reflected God," he told Lucado, "to the nurses, the doctors, my friends. Who knows who needed to see God, but I did my best to make Him seen."[4]

My trial of fear and anxiety over flying pales in comparison to someone who is battling cancer. However, like Lucado's friend, I learned an unforgettable lesson about using our challenging circumstances to bring glory to Christ.

I had 16 hours over 16 flights to sit next to 16 different people. The first half of these trips I spent my time with my nose buried in the Bible; I was consumed by my anxiety and fear and it was all I could do to call out to the Lord for comfort. And He did give me comfort and peace. But then I realized that during my travels, I had never once told others of God's goodness and grace. The Lord clearly told me that He wanted that to change. God was calling me to be an airplane missionary.

The last two trips could not have been better. It was like God was "showing off" that He is ultimately in control. He abundantly blessed me with free airport shuttles and flights that arrived early to destinations. The Lord was telling me "Relax... and focus on the next blessing I have for you as you witness to others."

At first it was not easy to witness to my "plane buddies." I was at least proud of myself when I initiated a conversation with the person sitting next to me. But slowly the Lord gave me open doors or showed me ways to start conversations. My favorite line was to look out the window and say "Look how awesome those clouds are! Psalm 19 says that the Heavens declare the glory of God. How true, huh?" As I continued my attempts at witnessing, I felt ashamed that I didn't talk more or say the right things. The battle was raging in my mind again and the enemy was telling me that I was failing.

> *But if you suffer because you are a Christian, do not be ashamed. Praise God because you wear that name.*

- 1 Peter 4:16 (NCV)

The enemy's roar of fear and condemnation was finally silenced on my last flight home. I was still nervous boarding the plane, but I was confident in God's provision. And I was on a mission, I only had two more opportunities to share my faith. On the first leg of the trip, I was seated next to young man. I pulled out all the stops, trying everything I could think of to talk to him about God, church, and Jesus. He brushed off every attempt to talk to him about spiritual things, though he had no problem talking to me about his job or sports!

As I waited for my connecting flight, the final leg of my trip home, I felt defeated that I hadn't seemed to get through to him. I was ready to call it quits and just rest on my last flight, especially since I had only had 3 hours of sleep the night before. But in obedience I said "Lord... who's next? One last one... let's do this together. Who will you have me talk to now?"

I boarded the plane one more time and submitted my anxiety to Him. I sat and immediately pulled out my Bible and had it open and ready. It was a full flight. As more and more people filled the plane, I had no fear, just anticipation of who would sit next to me. Finally, the plane doors closed and realization struck: the flight was full and I was the only person with an empty seat next to me. I breathed a sigh of relief as I laid back and looked out the window. In His mercy, the Lord had given me rest. As the plane took off for home, I heard very clearly "well done, good and faithful servant".

To God alone be the glory! I am a different person today because of my submission to Him in trials such as these.

His faithfulness led to my deliverance from the consuming sin of fear and worry. However, that does not mean that I do not still struggle (sometimes daily) with worry and anxiety. But it no longer consumes me. It no longer defines who I am... Jesus defines who I am!

If you are consumed by a besetting sin such as vanity, pride, overindulgence, worry or fear, know that Jesus will deliver you. He is a pain taker and chain breaker. And He will not leave you on your own to struggle and "figure it out yourself."

Even in victory, there can still be moments of struggle. But the struggle doesn't define who we are... the struggle helps us define who our King is. And if you allow Him, He will be everything you need in the midst of the trial. By setting your eyes on Him, He will pull you closer and closer, until His embrace floods your heart with such peace and joy that you wonder why you were anxious in the first place.

However, to get to that place in your walk with Him, it takes an intentional investment of time and effort, which is what we'll look at in the next chapter.

CHAPTER 13

The Bread of Life

For in Him we live and move and have our being...

– Acts 17:28

That is one of my all-time favorite verses. What a wonderful reminder of who my focus should be on! With that verse in mind, let's look at another amazing passage:

I once thought these things were valuable, but now I consider them worthless because of what Christ has done. Yes, everything else is worthless when compared with the infinite value of knowing Christ Jesus my Lord. For his sake I have discarded everything else, counting it all as garbage, so that I could gain Christ and become one with him. I no longer count on my own righteousness through obeying the law; rather, I become righteous through faith in Christ. For God's way of making us right with himself depends on faith. I want to know Christ and experience the mighty power that raised him from the dead. I want to suffer with him, sharing in his death, so that one way or another I will experience the resurrection from the dead!

- Philippians 3:7-11 (NLT)

Through Christ we've been set free from our bondage to sin. We've been ransomed, our sin-debt has been paid and the penalty of spiritual death has been lifted. And we've been justified - which means God sees us "just as if we have never sinned." It is because of this that Paul can claim: "Yes, everything is worthless when compared with the infinite value of knowing Christ Jesus my Lord."

Like Paul, can we say that "for His sake I have discarded everything else, counting it all as garbage?" It's not so much of a stretch to apply this idea to what we eat. Whether we realize it or not, food takes a high priority in our lives. We plan our day around it. In fact, many of us plan our meals days and weeks in advance. We can honor Him by choosing what's best for us, both physically and spiritually.

Keeping in mind who we are made for and the price that was paid to redeem us, let's remember what Jesus said about fueling our bodies:

> And Jesus said to them, "I am the bread of life. He who comes to Me shall never hunger, and he who believes in Me shall never thirst.
>
> - John 6:35

Whatever our need is, whether to feel worthy, loved, beautiful, comforted, desired, or at peace; these can be fulfilled in Christ. He is our ultimate source of nourishment. And therefore, He should be our ultimate desire.

Do we diligently plan our day around spending time in the Word and spending time with the only true source of sustenance?

To make meals for our family, it takes an investment of planning, preparing and presenting. We plan the meals for the week. We prepare by shopping and chopping and crock-potting. And we don't just throw the result in a pile on a plate, we present it in a way that is appealing and appetizing.

What if we were to take the same approach with our time with the Lord?

Since He is our Sustainer, our source of true bread, the giver of every breath we breathe, shouldn't we be as intentional with the time we spend with Him as we are with the time that goes into our planning and preparing our meals?

Is your devotion time squeezed into the few minutes between waking and the chaos that ensues with the dawn of a new day? Perhaps grabbing your Bible, reading a chapter, and saying a quick prayer for your family and your busy day is all you can manage on most mornings.

That is OK. Better a few minutes spent in the Word and with the King than no time at all.

Yet, I want to encourage you to be as committed to spending time with Jesus as you are to spending time on meals.

What does that look like?

Well, we can use the same approach as we do with meals: plan, prepare, and present. Let's look at how this works in the next chapter.

CHAPTER 14

Plan, Prepare, Present

The devotional time that we spend with the Lord needs to be a high priority in our lives. I know you've heard that before, and if you're anything like me, you've tried multiple approaches to make it happen.

In this chapter, I want to give you a clear plan on how to implement a consistent and productive devotional time into your busy day. Like meal planning, we must plan, prepare and then present.

Plan

I wish I could say that if you ask nicely, the Lord would align the cosmos to allow you to have an hour of uninterrupted, peaceful and fruitful devotional time each morning. However, that is not the case. We need to plan. Step one of that plan is to present your intentions to the Lord and ASK!

If it is a struggle to find time to meet with Him, then tell Him you need help! Ask Him to help you wake up an hour earlier. Ask Him to help you prioritize the rest of your morning to free up some time. Ask Him which devotional books should accompany your regular Bible reading. Ask Him! He promises to provide the things we need, and what we need most is Him!

To make room for devotional time with our King, you may find that something needs to be sacrificed from your regular schedules. Perhaps it means less sleep. Or maybe it means sacrificing time that you would normally spend reading for fun, playing video games, watching TV or movies, doing crafts, or even preparing meals. It's not easy to sacrifice. However, I guarantee that the time you spend with the Lord will pay itself back tenfold - physically, spiritually and emotionally.

Therefore, planning is critical. We set the alarm a little earlier. We tell our family members that this time is not to be interrupted. And we stick to it.

We also need to know how exactly we'll be spending the time. I suggest three components: Bible reading, prayer, and a study book.

If you don't have one already, I highly suggest a "read through the Bible in a year" Bible. These Bibles include a daily reading composed of a chapter or two from the Old Testament, Psalms, Proverbs, and the New Testament. By sticking with the plan, you'll read through the whole Bible in a year.

I also recommend a study book of some kind. This can be Bible study, a devotional book, a Bible commentary, or a book that edifies and encourages.

Bonus: For a list of some of my favorite and treasured books, see the Recommended Resources at the end of this book.

And then there is prayer. Prayer can be tricky for many people. If you need a little help, you can use the ACTS format. This will be covered in the next chapter.

Prepare

So, we've made some plans for our devotion time. We've identified a time slot, gathered the resources we'll use (Bible, devotionals, prayer journals, etc.), and now we need to prepare.

First, we need to prepare a place. It needs to be somewhere comfortable (but not so comfortable that you drift off to sleep during prayer!). It needs to be somewhere that is free from distractions. And it needs to be somewhere quiet.

Sounds like quite a wish list, doesn't it? It may take a little work, a little arranging, and a little cajoling and bribing of other family members, but you can do it. You can set aside a place and dedicate some time to be with your King. It is so worth it!

I know some women who put a recliner in their bedroom. That way they can get up first thing in the morning, grab their coffee and then retreat to their room, away from the business and noise of the rest of the house.

Other women have an office or den they can use. Maybe it is just the living room couch. Perhaps if your neighborhood is quiet enough, you can sit on the porch.

Wherever it is, stake your claim and make sure the rest of your household knows not to disturb you during your devotional time.

Present

I have a weakness for watching cooking shows. The Food Network is one of my guilty pleasures. I love watching the shows where competing chefs are eliminated one by one at each round. Chefs frequently lose points over presentation.

It happens like this: the clock shows there is only a few seconds left for the competitors to get their food on a plate and present it to the judges. The chefs who haven't managed their time wisely end up tossing the food on the plate with no time to arrange it and make it look as appetizing as possible.

Let's not do the same thing with the time that we give to the Lord. We should present ourselves to the Lord in such a way as to show we are serious about meeting with Him. We should show Him we recognize the blessing and the privilege it is to meet with the King of Kings.

To do this, we need to prepare our heart and minds before we present them to Him.

I don't know about you, but I have found that it is awful hard to concentrate on reading the Bible if I am consumed with thoughts of what the day will bring. Let's face it, as women, there is a lot on our plates and it can be very difficult to "turn off" our active minds so that we can focus on the Lord.

So, what can we do? Some women find it helpful to do a little worship first. This could mean using a worship CD or streaming some worship songs on your phone. You don't need to necessarily sing out loud, you can close your eyes and "sing" along with the songs in your head.

Maybe you can clear your head with a quick walk around the block, or a few minutes on the treadmill to get your blood flowing. Perhaps a hot shower and a quick bowl of oatmeal would do the trick.

Whatever you do, avoid anything that can add to your distractions or end up taking away time that you have set aside to spend with the Lord. Don't get up and check your email first, or turn on the news, or even check Facebook. We are trying to clear your mind of distractions, not add to them!

Maybe you have already discovered a good method to prepare yourself before starting your devotion time. If not, experiment with a few of the suggestions or try something else - just don't expect to pick up your Bible and be able to dive right in without a little prep time - not if you want a fruitful and tender time with your Savior.

Oh, and ask Him! Start with a quick prayer and ask the Lord to quiet your heart and mind, to minimize distractions, to open your spiritual eyes and ears, and to give you a sensitivity to what He wants you to hear from Him during your time spent together.

Present yourself to the Lord in such a way that you are ready to listen and respond to His prompting through the Holy Spirit. And come with expectation, He always shows up and His Word never returns void - it's our responsibility to come ready to hear from Him.

The ACTS Prayer

Is your prayer life feeling a little dry? We hear teachings on prayer all the time. We know the value of it, and we desperately want to do it. So why is it such a struggle? Why does it feel more like a chore than a privilege?

I want to share a simple method for structuring your prayer time for maximum benefit. Maybe you've heard of it before. When I first learned it, and began to implement it, I couldn't believe how it transformed my prayer time. I went from bringing God a laundry-list of requests to having an intimate time of talking with my Savior.

It is called the ACTS method of prayer. ACTS stands for:

A - Adoration

C - Confession

T - Thanksgiving

S – Supplication

Let's look at each step in more detail.

Adoration

Start by adoring God. He is so worthy of our worship! Therefore, to get our mind and heart in the right place for prayer, we should start by acknowledging and recognizing who we are praying to.

What does this look like? Essentially, we need start by putting things in perspective.

We are the creation, He is the Creator.

We are sinners saved by grace, He is sinless and Holy.

We are weak, He is strong.

We struggle and fail, He is faithful and unchanging.

You can even start your prayer with a simple song that adores the Lord. I am sure you have some favorite worship songs, and any song that speaks of God's attributes and encourages us to worship and adore Him will work well. And you can always fall back on the classic, "Father, I Adore You." Here are the lyrics if you are not familiar with it:

Father, I adore You.
I lay my heart before You.
How I love You.
Spirit, I adore You.
I lay my heart before You.
How I love You.
Jesus, I adore You.
I lay my heart before You.
How I love You.

If you've never heard it before, you can find it on YouTube with a quick search.

A daily recognition of who God is has been an incredible help to me in my battle against food cravings. One afternoon I was in a funky mood. I had a bad day at work and I really wanted some cookies. I bought a bag of gluten free chocolate chip cookies and I ate one. Then I ate another. Then another. I knew this action of cookie indulgence was not beneficial to me - and each time I reached for another cookie I felt that "nudge" saying "no Erica, you don't need that." I think we've all felt that Holy Spirit "nudge" at some point.

As I reached for that fourth cookie, I could feel myself intentionally ignoring that nudge and saying "No, I really want this cookie!" At that moment, I very clearly heard a response I will never forget "Who do you think you are saying 'no' to, Erica?" Instantly I realized I was saying "no" to my Creator and King - the all-powerful, all knowing and awesome God. I was ashamed. I dared to say "no" to Him over a cookie, even after already having three of them! Ever since then, I've been taking the "adoration" part of prayer very seriously. Reminding myself daily of who God is, and who I am by comparison, helps me to follow His design for my body.

Confession

After getting our hearts prepared by adoring God, then we move into a time of confession. Confession is simply acknowledging our sin before God. We aren't revealing anything the Lord doesn't already know. Confession isn't for His sake, it is for ours. Our sin breaks His heart. We need to recognize that fact and understand the full weight of our sin. And we need to understand the price that was paid to forgive and remove our sin.

Even though His amazing grace never runs dry, we can't be flippant about sin. It is serious. It is infectious. And it is deadly. That is why we must confess it.

> *If we confess our sins, He is faithful and just to forgive us our sins and to cleanse us from all unrighteousness.*
>
> *- 1 John 1:9*

Wow. Despite our unfaithfulness, He is faithful. When sin mars us like mud and filth, He cleanses us.

Want to know something else amazing? Something that drops me to my knees in awe every time I think of it?

When we ask the Lord to forgive us, you know what His response is?

"I already did."

Your sins were forgiven on the cross. Every sin. Every single sin you ever did and ever will do. They've been forgiven! Each and every one of them!

Your debt has been paid. Your slate has been wiped clean.

We don't confess so that we can be forgiven. He already did that. We confess to recognize and acknowledge that we've broken His law and broken His heart.

We confess so that He can cleanse. There is nothing like starting the day with a heart that has been cleansed and refreshed through confession!

Thanksgiving

> *We adore, we confess, then we give thanks.*
> *Oh, give thanks to the Lord, for He is good!*
> *For His mercy endures forever.*
>
> *- 1 Chronicles 16:34*

Regardless of our present circumstances in life, we still have a lot to be thankful for. He has blessed us in so many amazing ways! Spend this time recognizing His blessing and provision in your life.

> *I will praise the Lord according to His righteousness,*
> *And will sing praise to the name of the Lord Most High.*
>
> *- Psalm 7:17*

Thank Him for His faithfulness, His love, His kindness and generosity. Thank Him for your family, your house, your job, and your spouse. Thank Him for the gift of His Son and for the presence of the Holy Spirit in your life. Thank Him for walking with you through the trials you are facing, and the trials you have already overcome. Thank Him for His promise to never leave nor forsake.

Once you've spent time adoring the Lord and confessing your sin, you will naturally be left with a heart of thankfulness. Gratitude will begin to bubble forth. Perhaps a trickle at first, but once you begin to comprehend all that He has done for you, your trickle of gratitude will become a flood!

Supplication

> *Be anxious for nothing, but in everything by prayer and supplication,*
> *with thanksgiving, let your requests be made known to God.*
>
> *- Philippians 4:6*

This is what most people think of when they hear the word "pray." For many people, prayer is a time of making requests of God. But as we have seen, prayer can be and should be so much more than that. The reason I love this ACTS model of prayer is that it puts the least emphasis on our requests.

Many times, I start my prayer time with what I need from God (or what I think I need at least). I rattle off a "shopping list" of requests and worries. However, I have always found that when I start my prayer time with adoration, confession and thanksgiving - by the time I get to supplication, suddenly there is a lot less that I ask Him for. When we take the time to put things in proper perspective, our request list shrinks as we realize and recognize God's plan, provision, and providence in our lives.

With that said though, don't be bashful. Don't hold back. Ask for the little things. Ask for the big things. You're talking to the God who spoke the world into existence out of nothing! Who else can we take our concerns over cancer reports and job losses to?

Yet, He is also the God who knows every hair on our head - He knows us intimately. So even the little requests can be brought before Him. He is a loving Father and there is a special place in His heart for His daughters.

CHAPTER 16

There Is Grace

The next time you eat in response to a strong emotion, don't lament your lack of willpower. Research shows that treating yourself gently may help you stave off future bouts of emotional eating.

In 2007, researchers at Wake Forest University asked female subjects to taste test doughnuts. Half of the women weren't given any special instruction. The other half were first given a lesson in self-compassion. The tester said something like, "I hope you won't be too hard on yourself. Everyone in the study eats this stuff." The result: Those who received the "be kind to yourself" or self-compassionate mandate ultimately ate fewer sweets.[3]

Therefore, treat yourself firmly but lovingly. That is how our Father treats us: he corrects with a gentle grace.

The enemy would love to keep us in bondage to our failures and shortcomings. He would love to rub our failures in our face and stir up anger, resentment and bitter feelings in our heart.

He is a two-faced sneak! First, he will tempt us. He knows just what buttons to push, whether it is directed at our willpower over junk food or some other area we are struggling with in our lives. He comes tempting and cajoling, enticing and alluring. But when we

CREATED TO CRAVE • 67

succumb, when we stumble and fall - suddenly he yells, "Aha! You are worthless! You couldn't even keep from eating another helping of ice cream. You have no self-control. You are going to gain 100 pounds!"

He tempts, and then when we fall, he condemns. He kicks us when we are down. There is only one cure.

Grace.

Just like any good parent who picks up their child when they fail at something, our Heavenly Father comes alongside, picks us up and says, "It is OK, my dear daughter. Try again. I bring no condemnation. Lean on me. When you are weak, I am strong. I love you dearly. Don't forget, you are fearfully and wonderfully made, by my very hands. And nothing can separate you from my love!"

The condemnation from the enemy or even the anger we feel towards ourselves for failing can be answered by this amazing promise from our Savior:

> *A soft answer turns away wrath, but a harsh word stirs up anger.*
>
> *- Proverbs 15:1*

Let Jesus' soft word to you expel any anger from the enemy.

We all stumble. We all fail. We must learn from our mistake, set our eyes on our Savior, and move on!

> *Not that I have already attained, or am already perfected; but I press on, that I may lay hold of that for which Christ Jesus has also laid hold of me. Brethren, I do not count myself to have apprehended; but one thing I do, forgetting those things which are behind and reaching forward to those things which are ahead, I press toward the goal for the prize of the upward call of God in Christ Jesus.*
>
> *- Philippians 3:12-14*

The amazing thing about our Lord is that He will reward us with crowns for being faithful and obedient in the race He has set before us. But even more amazing is that He is the one who will strengthen and enable us to run that race. We are not doing this alone, and this race is not designed to be done in our own strength.

Don't forget that we each run our own race. Don't look at your sister in Christ. She is running a different race, that is her race. You need to run your race.

And never forget that we don't run alone.

> *I will never leave you nor forsake you.*
>
> *- Hebrews 13:5*

Christ goes before us, all we need to do is set our eyes on Him and we will make it to the finish line.

One of my favorite worship songs goes like this:

> *I know who goes before me*
> *I know who stands behind*
> *The God of angel armies*
> *Is always by my side*
> *The one who reigns forever*
> *He is a friend of mine*
> *The God of angel armies*
> *Is always by my side*
> *And nothing formed against me shall stand*
> *You hold the whole world in your hands*
> *I'm holding on to your promises*
> *You are faithful, You are faithful* [5]
>
> *Whom Shall I Fear By Chris Tomlin*

He is so amazingly faithful, isn't He? It boggles my mind that the God of all creation would call us friend, that He would care about our struggles. He does! And He loves us with a passionate, unquenchable love!

CHAPTER 17

Simplify Your Life

Feeling "burned-out" can easily lead to emotional eating. Researchers found that women who were overwhelmed on the job or at home were significantly more likely to use food as a source of comfort and relief. So, no, you aren't alone in this struggle.

> *But seek first the kingdom of God and His righteousness, and all these things shall be added to you.*
>
> *- Matthew 6:33*

Sounds nice, right? But what does seeking Him first actually look like in practice?

Here are some practical ideas to help you win the battle against business:

Simplify Your House

Managing your household can be a huge source of stress, especially if you are married and have kids.

Start by decluttering the house. Have a yard sale and get rid of as much stuff as your family will let you!

Then get bins for the remaining stuff. Put one in each of the kid's bedrooms and one in the play area or living room. Teach the kids that they must put their toys back in the bins when they are done playing with them. Enforce it! If they don't follow the rule, the toy gets taken away for a time.

Enlist your husband and kids with the laundry, dishes, or cleaning schedule. Set up a "chore chart" and keep track of progress. Reward your family when they do a job well done.

Simplify Your Meals

Are there certain forms of junk food that tempt you more than others? If so, stop buying them at the grocery store. Yes, the rest of your family might be bummed, but you can explain that this is a way they can support you.

Plan your meals in advance. Stressful days will more likely lead to quick meals that are full of unneeded calories (fat/sugar) and processed foods. Only buy foods on a well thought out and budgeted list. Use your crockpot or make freezer meals for quick defrosting during the week (see Appendix 1 for ideas and recipes).

Here are a few good "rules of thumb" you can follow:

- Eat sweet treats only on the weekends.
- Don't eat after 7:00 PM and don't eat while watching TV.
- Kids rules apply to adults too - you must eat all your veggies before you can leave the table!
- Get a smaller dinner plate to avoid overeating by limiting yourself to smaller portions.

- Chew your foods completely. Chew until you can no longer distinguish what food you ate. You shouldn't be able to tell whether you have oatmeal or steak in your mouth. This slower eating will help reduce overeating and aid in digestion, helping you to feel fuller, faster!
- Eat breakfast like a queen, lunch like a princess, and dinner like a pauper. That means eat your carb-heavy, calorie-rich foods earlier in the day and eat mainly nutrient dense foods like veggies at the end of the day.

Bonus: These are just "quick and dirty" ideas you can begin to implement. For more detailed ideas, see the Recommended Resources section at the end of this book.

Simplify Your Schedule

This is a tricky one. You are probably involved in many "good" things like church ministries, kid's sports programs, school functions, work functions, and all manner of friends and family functions. But even "good" things can cause stress and may not be for the best in the long run.

Are there some things that you can get help with or delegate to others? Are we willing to relinquish control? Are we ready to prioritize and then minimize?

The trick is to learn to say "no." Do it gracefully, but start declining more responsibility. Obviously, you'll need to spend some time in prayer and get the Lord involved in your decision making in this area. It may just be a busy season in your life. However, when your sanity is on the line and it is affecting other areas of your life, especially your relationship with the Lord, then it is time to cut back!

CHAPTER 18

Remember Our Destination

For our citizenship is in heaven, from which we also eagerly wait for the Savior, the Lord Jesus Christ, who will transform our lowly body that it may be conformed to His glorious body, according to the working by which He is able even to subdue all things to Himself.

- Philippians 3:20-21

Right now we are fighting a war against things that want to pull us away from victory in Christ. Emotional eating can consume us. Stress, hormones, food sensitivities, anxieties, feelings of unworthiness, and so much more - can make us turn to food or other poor choices.

Someday every struggle will be over and we will be standing in the presence of our Lord and Savior. We'll have new bodies (perfect bodies!), but at that time we won't care about our weight, how we look or how we feel. Instead, we will be overwhelmed with His power, majesty, and love for us.

Until that day though, we'll continue the battle against our fleshly desires and emotional responses. As we learn to submit to Him, as we learn to surrender our cravings and give Him full permission to use our lives for His glory, we'll gain the victory.

We'll overcome the struggles, we'll conquer the temptations, and we'll find that our desires have been redirected and fulfilled by the only One who can bring complete satisfaction, endless joy and lasting peace.

Take heart dear sister! He loves you with an unconditional love and He has an amazing plan for your life.

> *And I am certain that God, who began the good work within you, will continue his work until it is finally finished on the day when Christ Jesus returns.*
>
> *- Philippians 1:6 (NLT)*

NOTE FROM THE AUTHOR

Thank you so much for reading! I hope and pray you were blessed by this book.

If you enjoyed the book, I'd greatly appreciate a positive review on Amazon.

I'd also love to hear from you if you have feedback or questions. To contact me, visit my website:

www.ericacallahan.com

Appendix 1 – Who I Am In Christ

As you read through this list of scriptures, you may find some hard to believe to be true about you. But they are. All of them! They are taken from the Word of God. God's Word is infallible, He has preserved it supernaturally and the promises found within it are true and dependable.

You are a child of God. You are accepted. You are secure. You are significant.

Read through the list slowly. And don't forget, these statements about you are true at this very moment. These aren't promises reserved for heaven or for a more spiritually mature version of you. These promises are true today!

For a printable version of this list ("Who I Am In Christ"), go to the Resources page on my website: www.ericacallahan.com

I Am Accepted...

I am God's child.
- John 1:12

As a disciple, I am a friend of Jesus Christ.
- John 15:15

I have been justified.
- Romans 5:1

I am united with the Lord, and I am one with Him in spirit.
- 1 Corinthians 6:17

I have been bought with a price and I belong to God.
- 1 Corinthians 6:19-20

I am a member of Christ's body.
- 1 Corinthians 12:27

I have been chosen by God and adopted as His child.
- Ephesians 1:3-8

*I have been redeemed and forgiven of **all** my sins.*
- Colossians 1:13-14

I am complete in Christ.
- Colossians 2:9-10

I have direct access to the throne of grace through Jesus Christ.
- Hebrews 4:14-16

I Am Secure...

I am free from condemnation.
- Romans 8:1-2

I am assured that God works for my good in all circumstances.
- Romans 8:28

I am free from any condemnation brought against me and I cannot be separated from the love of God. - Romans 8:31-39

I have been established, anointed and sealed by God.
- 2 Corinthians 1:21-22

I am hidden with Christ in God.
- Colossians 3:1-4

I am confident that God will complete the good work He started in me. - Philippians 1:6

I am a citizen of heaven.
- Philippians 3:20

I have not been given a spirit of fear but of power, love and a sound mind. - 2 Timothy 1:7

I am born of God and the evil one cannot touch me.
- 1 John 5:18

I Am Significant...

I am a branch of Jesus Christ, the true vine, and a channel of His life. - John 15:5

I have been chosen and appointed to bear fruit.
- John 15:16

I am God's temple.
- 1 Corinthians 3:1

I am a minister of reconciliation for God.
- 2 Corinthians 5:17-21

I am seated with Jesus Christ in the heavenly realm.
- Ephesians 2:6

I am God's workmanship.
- Ephesians 2:10

I may approach God with freedom and confidence.
- Ephesians 3:12

I can do all things through Christ, who strengthens me.
- Philippians 4:13

Source: Anderson, N. (n.d.). Who I Am In Christ. Retrieved September 23, 2015, from https://www.ficm.org/handy-links/#!/who-i-am-in-christ

If you perpetually struggle with fear, anxiety and worry like I do, then I encourage you to keep these scriptures close at hand.

I like to write a verse on a sticky-note and keep them around the house where I'll constantly see them. I keep the list of scriptures in my purse for easy reference. I try to memorize as many of them as I can. Doing these things has radically changed my outlook when I am faced with a situation that would otherwise cause me to be filled with fear and anxiety. The Truth of God's Word is powerful!

Worry and Anxiety

Matthew 6:25-27 - "Therefore I tell you, do not be anxious about your life, what you will eat or what you will drink, nor about your body, what you will put on. Is not life more than food, and the body more than clothing? Look at the birds of the air: they neither sow nor reap nor gather into barns, and yet your heavenly Father feeds them. Are you not of more value than they? And which of you by being anxious can add a single hour to his span of life?"

Matthew 6:34 - "Therefore do not be anxious about tomorrow, for tomorrow will be anxious for itself. Sufficient for the day is its own trouble."

Matthew 11:28-30 - "Come to me, all who labor and are heavy laden, and I will give you rest. Take my yoke upon you, and learn from me, for I am gentle and lowly in heart, and you will find rest for your souls. For my yoke is easy, and my burden is light."

Luke 12:25 - "And which of you by being anxious can add a single hour to his span of life?"

John 14:27 - "Peace I leave with you; my peace I give to you. Not as the world gives do I give to you. Let not your hearts be troubled, neither let them be afraid."

Proverbs 12:25 - "Anxiety in a man's heart weighs him down, but a good word makes him glad."

Philippians 4:6-7 - "Do not be anxious about anything, but in everything by prayer and supplication with thanksgiving let your requests be made known to God. And the peace of God, which surpasses all understanding, will guard your hearts and your minds in Christ Jesus."

1 Peter 5:7 - "Casting all your anxieties on Him, because He cares for you."

Peace and Purpose

Colossians 3:15 - "And let the peace of Christ rule in your hearts, to which indeed you were called in one body. And be thankful."

2 Thessalonians 3:16 - "Now may the Lord of peace himself give you peace at all times in every way. The Lord be with you all."

Psalm 55:22 - "Cast your burden on the LORD, and he will sustain you; he will never permit the righteous to be moved."

Isaiah 26:3 - "You will keep him in perfect peace, whose mind is stayed on You, because he trusts in You."

Acts 17:28 - "For in Him we live, and move and have our being..."

Isaiah 58:10-11 - "If you pour out for the hungry and satisfy the desire of the afflicted, then shall your light rise in the darkness and your gloom be as the noonday. And the Lord will guide you continually and satisfy your desire in scorched places and make your bones strong; and you shall be like a watered garden, like a spring of water, whose waters do not fail."

Psalm 46:10 - "Be still, and know that I am God. I will be exalted among the nations, I will be exalted in the earth!"

Proverbs 3:5-6 - "Trust in the LORD with all your heart, and do not lean on your own understanding. In all your ways acknowledge him, and he will make straight your paths."

Do Not Fear

Psalm 23:4 - "Even though I walk through the valley of the shadow of death, I will fear no evil, for you are with me; your rod and your staff, they comfort me."

Isaiah 43:1-3 - "But now thus says the LORD, he who created you, O Jacob, he who formed you, O Israel: "Fear not, for I have redeemed you; I have called you by name, you are mine. When you pass through the waters, I will be with you; and through the rivers, they shall not overwhelm you; when you walk through fire you shall not be burned, and the flame shall not consume you. For I am the LORD your God, the Holy One of Israel, your Savior."

Hebrews 13:6 - "So we can confidently say, 'The Lord is my helper; I will not fear; what can man do to me?'"

Psalm 56:3 - "When I am afraid, I put my trust in you."

Psalm 121:1-2 - "I lift up my eyes to the hills. From where does my help come? My help comes from the LORD, who made heaven and earth."

1 Corinthians 10:13 - "No temptation has overtaken you that is not common to man. God is faithful, and he will not let you be tempted beyond your ability, but with the temptation he will also provide the way of escape, that you may be able to endure it."

Romans 8:31 - "What then shall we say to these things? If God is for us, who can be against us?"

APPENDIX 3- SIMPLE AND HEALTHY RECIPES

Planning and cooking healthy (and delicious!) meals for our family each week can be a huge time investment and a source of constant stress. It doesn't have to be though!

One of the best suggestions I can give is to use your crockpot. Lots! I cook at least 4 meals every week in the crockpot. And my family loves them! They are easy to prepare and typically much healthier than other meals – especially meals that are prepared when we are pressed for time.

Crockpot 365 Blog

www.ayearofslowcooking.com

Contains crockpot recipes with simple ingredients (many are gluten free) for every day of the year.

60+ Healthy Freezer Meals

http://thrivinghomeblog.com/healthy-recipes-index/healthy-freezer-meals-recipes/

Blog with how to prepare and freeze meals, tips on what types of storage containers to use and over 60 recipes.

Healthy Recipes Kids Might Love

http://www.foodnetwork.com/recipes/photos/our-best-healthy-recipes-for-kids-and-families.html

Food Network's top picks for healthy and fun foods for kids.

Super Healthy Kids

http://www.superhealthykids.com/healthy-kids-recipes/

Blog with lots of fun kid-friendly, healthy meal and dessert ideas.

Vegan Recipe Websites

http://www.101cookbooks.com/vegan_recipes/

http://ohmyveggies.com/category/vegan-recipes/page/2/

Two websites with lots of veggie-based recipes.

Healthy Party Appetizers

http://www.cookingchanneltv.com/recipes/low-calorie-appetizers-and-party-foods.html

Cooking Channel's best, healthiest party foods.

Below is a simple good diary that you can use to keep track what you eat and how you feel throughout the day. For a printable version, check out the Resources page on my website: www.ericacallahan.com

Daily Food Tracker

Today's Date: _____

Time	Food	Amount	I am feeling...	I am doing...
			☺ ☹	
			☺ ☹	
			☺ ☹	
			☺ ☹	
			☺ ☹	
			☺ ☹	
			☺ ☹	
			☺ ☹	
			☺ ☹	
			☺ ☹	

Amount of Sleep Last Night: _____

Energy Level Today: _____

Water Intake Today: _____

Bibliography

1 - Anderson, N. (n.d.). Who I Am In Christ. Retrieved September 23, 2015, from https://www.ficm.org/handy-links/#!/who-i-am-in-christ

2 - Wiersbe, W. (1979) "The Strategy of Satan: How to Detect and Defeat Him." Mass Market Paperback, Fleming H Revell Company.

3 - Adams, CE & Leary MR. (2007) "Promoting Self Compassionate Attitudes Towards Eating Among Restrictive and Guilty Eaters". Journal of Social and Clinical Psychology. Vol. 26, No. 10, p. 1120-1144.

4 - Lucado, Max. It's Not about Me: Rescue from the Life We Thought Would Make Us Happy. Nashville: Integrity, 2004. 125-26. Print.

5 - Tomlin, Chris. Whom Shall I Fear. Burning Lights. Chris Tomlin. EMI/Sixsteprecords/Sparrow Records, 2013. MP3.

Made in the USA
Middletown, DE
15 August 2018